STIFF F _____
SYNDROME DIET

Complete Guide To Understanding And Thriving
With A Personalized Diet Plan, Including Meal
Plans, Recipes, And Lifestyle Strategies For
Optimal Health And Well-Being.

Dr. Holmgren Alfred

Disclaimer

The information in this book, "Stiff Person Syndrome Diet: With Expert Guidance," is intended for informational purposes only and is not intended to be a substitute for professional medical advice, diagnosis, or treatment. If you have any questions about a medical condition, always seek the advice of your physician or other qualified health provider. Never disregard or delay seeking professional medical advice because of something you have read in

The author of this book, is not a medical professional and does not claim to be one. The content of this book is based on research, personal experience, and expert opinions gathered from various sources. While efforts have been made to ensure the accuracy of the information provided, the author makes no representations or warranties of any kind, express or implied, regarding the completeness, accuracy, reliability, suitability, or availability concerning the

The author does not endorse or recommend any individuals, products, websites, organizations, or other names mentioned in this book; all such references are provided for informational purposes only and should not be interpreted as an endorsement or recommendation. The author disclaims any liability for any loss or damage arising from the use of information or reliance on any recommendations mentioned in this book.

Furthermore, individual dietary demands and responses to dietary changes may vary, so it is critical to check with a certified healthcare expert before making any significant changes to your diet or lifestyle, especially if you have a medical condition like Stiff Person Syndrome.

By reading this book, you agree that the author is not liable for any repercussions that may arise from the use of the information provided herein. You also understand that you are solely responsible for any actions you take based on the information contained in this book.

ABOUT THIS BOOK.

Stiff Person Syndrome Diet: With Expert Guidance" is an indispensable resource tailored to empower individuals navigating the complexities of Stiff Person Syndrome (SPS). This comprehensive guide transcends mere dietary advice, offering a holistic approach to managing SPS symptoms with expert insight and practical strategies.

The book's central premise is that diet plays a critical role in mitigating SPS symptoms and optimizing overall well-being. It illuminates the symbiotic relationship between nutrition and SPS progression, underscoring the profound impact of dietary choices on symptom management. Through meticulous exploration, readers gain a nuanced understanding of essential nutrients, foods to embrace, and those to avoid, tailored specifically for individuals dealing with SPS.

With a focus on individualized dietary needs, readers are guided through the process of crafting personalized meal plans that strike a delicate balance between nourishment and enjoyment. What distinguishes this book is its pragmatic approach to translating nutritional science into actionable steps. From assessing dietary requirements to navigating meal preparation and cooking techniques, the book offers a roadmap to culinary empowerment for SPS patients and their caregivers.

In addition to dietary insights, the book addresses the myriad challenges inherent in managing SPS, ranging from coping with food intolerances to navigating social situations. It emphasizes the importance of holistic lifestyle strategies, advocating for the integration of physical activity, stress management techniques, and optimal sleep hygiene into daily routines to supplement dietary efforts.

Furthermore, "Stiff Person Syndrome Diet: With Expert Guidance" does not leave readers stranded after the final page, but rather serves as a gateway to a vibrant community of support, offering access to online communities, recommended resources, and professional nutritional counseling. By fostering a sense of camaraderie and empowerment, the book extends its impact beyond mere information dissemination, fostering a culture of resilience and collective empowerment among SPS patients.

CHAPTER 1

UNDERSTANDING STIFF PERSON SYNDROME

Introduction to Stiff Person Syndrome:

Stiff Person Syndrome (SPS) is a rare neurological disorder characterized by progressive muscle stiffness and rigidity, leading to significant disability and impairment in mobility. Since its first description in the medical literature in the 1950s, researchers have been striving to understand its underlying mechanisms and develop effective treatment strategies. SPS primarily affects the central nervous system, specifically the brain and spinal cord.

Causes And Risk Factors:

The exact cause of Stiff Person Syndrome remains unknown, but it is believed to be an autoimmune disorder in which the body's immune system mistakenly attacks its cells, particularly those involved in regulating muscle tone. Genetic predisposition may also play a role, as certain genetic variations have been associated with an increased risk of developing SPS. Furthermore, environmental factors such as infections or physical trauma may trigger the onset.

Symptoms And Diagnostics:

Individuals with Stiff Person Syndrome (SPS) may experience muscle spasms, involuntary contractions, and exaggerated startle responses, also known as "startle attacks," which can further impair mobility. Muscle stiffness and rigidity, which often begin in the axial muscles of the trunk and spread to the limbs, can be continuous or episodic, with exacerbations triggered by stress, sudden movements, or emotional distress.

Treatment Alternatives and Management Strategies:

Currently, there is no cure for Stiff Person Syndrome, and treatment primarily focuses on managing symptoms and improving quality of life. Medications such as benzodiazepines, muscle relaxants, and anti-seizure drugs may help alleviate muscle stiffness and spasms in some individuals. Intravenous immunoglobulin (IVIG) therapy and plasma exchange have also shown promise in reducing disease activity and improving motor function by modulating the immune response. Physical therapy and occupational therapy are essential components of SPS management, as they can help maintain flexibility, strength, and range of motion, as well as develop strategies to cope with activities of daily living. In severe cases where conservative measures are ineffective, surgical interventions such as intrathecal baclofen pump placement or deep brain stimulation may be considered to manage refractory symptoms. Additionally, lifestyle modifications such as stress management techniques, adequate rest, and avoiding triggers that exacerbate symptoms can help individuals with SPS better cope with their condition and optimize their overall health and well-being. Ongoing research efforts aimed at elucidating the underlying pathophysiology of SPS and developing targeted therapies hold promise for improving outcomes and quality of life for affected individuals in the future.

CHAPTER 2

THE IMPORTANCE OF DIET IN STIFF PERSON SYNDROME MANAGEMENT

Understanding the intricate relationship between diet and Stiff Person Syndrome (SPS) is essential for developing effective management strategies that can alleviate symptoms and improve the overall quality of life for people living with this condition. Among the various modalities used to treat and manage SPS, diet plays a critical role.

Diet In Managing SPS Symptoms.

Dietary interventions hold promise in managing the symptoms associated with Stiff Person Syndrome (SPS). While the exact mechanisms underlying the development and progression of SPS remain incompletely understood, emerging evidence suggests that certain dietary factors may influence symptom severity and frequency. For instance, dietary modifications aimed at reducing inflammation and oxidative stress have been proposed as potential strategies to mitigate the symptoms of SPS.

Additionally, dietary interventions targeting gut health and microbiota composition may also hold therapeutic potential in modulating immune function and reducing autoimmune-mediated symptoms characteristic of SPS. Moreover, dietary factors such as vitamin D status, omega-3 fatty acids, and antioxidants have been implicated in immune regulation and neuroprotection, which are relevant considerations in the management of SPS symptoms.

Thus, incorporating dietary interventions tailored to address specific nutritional needs and underlying pathophysiological mechanisms associated with SPS may offer promising avenues for symptom management and improved clinical outcomes.

Impact Of Nutrition On SPS Progression

Nutritional status and dietary patterns may exert profound effects on the progression and course of Stiff Person Syndrome (SPS). Emerging research suggests that nutritional factors play a role in modulating immune function, neuroinflammation, and neurotransmitter signaling pathways implicated in the pathogenesis of SPS.

For instance, deficiencies in certain vitamins and minerals, such as vitamin D, magnesium, and B vitamins, have been associated with immune dysregulation and neurologic dysfunction, which are hallmark features of SPS. Furthermore, imbalances in dietary fatty acids and alterations in gut microbiota composition have been linked to systemic inflammation and autoimmune processes implicated in SPS pathophysiology. Consequently, optimizing nutritional intake through dietary modifications and supplementation may help mitigate disease progression and attenuate symptom severity in individuals with SPS. Moreover, personalized nutrition approaches tailored to individual needs and metabolic profiles hold promise in optimizing nutrient status and supporting overall health and well-being in SPS patients.

By addressing nutritional imbalances and supporting key physiological pathways involved in SPS pathogenesis, nutrition-based interventions may complement conventional treatment modalities and contribute to more comprehensive management strategies for SPS.

Benefits Of A Well-Designed Diet Plan

Implementing a well-structured diet plan is paramount in managing Stiff Person Syndrome (SPS) effectively and promoting optimal health outcomes. A carefully designed diet plan can address specific nutritional needs, mitigate symptom severity, and support overall well-being in individuals with SPS. By focusing on nutrient-dense foods rich in vitamins, minerals, antioxidants, and essential fatty acids, a well-structured diet plan can help optimize immune function, reduce inflammation, and support neuroprotective mechanisms implicated in SPS pathophysiology. Additionally, a personalized diet plan can address individual dietary preferences, food intolerances, and metabolic imbalances, thereby enhancing compliance and long-term adherence to dietary interventions.

Moreover, incorporating lifestyle strategies such as stress management techniques, regular physical activity, and adequate sleep hygiene into the diet plan can further enhance its effectiveness in managing SPS symptoms and improving overall quality of life. Furthermore, ongoing monitoring and adjustment of the diet plan in response to changes in symptoms, nutritional status, and treatment outcomes are essential for optimizing therapeutic efficacy and achieving sustainable health benefits in individuals with SPS. In summary, a well-structured diet plan tailored to individual needs and preferences can serve as a cornerstone of comprehensive SPS management, offering significant potential for symptom relief, disease modulation, and improved overall well-being.

CHAPTER 3

NUTRITIONAL CONSIDERATIONS FOR STIFF PERSON'S SYNDROME

To manage Stiff Person Syndrome (SPS), a rare neurological disorder characterized by muscle stiffness and spasms, nutritional considerations are critical. Understanding the dietary needs of SPS patients involves careful attention to essential nutrients, foods to include and avoid, and the importance of hydration in maintaining optimal health and well-being.

Vitamin D, magnesium, calcium, and B vitamins are essential nutrients for SPS patients because they play vital roles in muscle function, nerve health, and bone density. Adequate intake of these nutrients can help alleviate muscle stiffness and spasms associated with SPS. Vitamin D, for example, supports immune function and may have anti-inflammatory properties.

Foods to include and avoid are central to designing a personalized diet plan for individuals with SPS. Including nutrient-dense foods such as fruits, vegetables, whole grains, lean proteins, and healthy fats can provide essential nutrients while supporting overall health. Fruits and vegetables are rich in vitamins, minerals, and antioxidants, which can help reduce inflammation and oxidative stress associated with SPS. Whole grains provide complex carbohydrates for sustained energy levels, while lean proteins supply amino acids necessary for muscle repair and function. Healthy fats from sources like nuts, seeds, and fatty fish offer anti-inflammatory properties and support brain health.

Conversely, certain foods may exacerbate symptoms or interfere with medication efficacy in SPS patients. These may include processed foods high in refined sugars and unhealthy fats, which can promote inflammation and worsen symptoms. Additionally, individuals with SPS may need to limit or avoid certain foods that trigger allergic or autoimmune responses, as these can potentially exacerbate symptoms and disrupt immune function. Therefore, a tailored approach to dietary management, focusing on nutrient-rich foods and minimizing potential triggers, is essential for optimizing health outcomes in SPS patients.

Hydration plays a critical role in supporting overall health and well-being, particularly for individuals with SPS. Adequate hydration is essential for maintaining proper muscle function, regulating body temperature, and supporting nutrient transport and waste removal. In SPS patients, muscle stiffness and spasms can increase fluid loss through sweating, potentially leading to dehydration if not adequately replenished. Dehydration can exacerbate symptoms such as fatigue, muscle cramps, and impaired cognitive function, making it essential for SPS patients to prioritize hydration as part of their daily routine. Optimal fluid intake varies depending on individual factors such as age, weight, activity level, and climate, but a general guideline is to consume at least 8-10 cups of water per day, adjusting intake as needed to maintain hydration status. In addition to water, hydrating fluids such as herbal teas, coconut water, and electrolyte-rich beverages can help replenish lost fluids and support hydration. Monitoring urine color and frequency can serve as indicators of hydration status, with pale yellow urine signifying adequate hydration. Therefore, integrating hydration strategies into the overall management plan for SPS can help optimize symptom management and improve the quality of life for affected individuals.

addressing nutritional considerations is integral to effectively managing Stiff Person Syndrome. Individuals with SPS can support overall health and well-being while managing symptoms more effectively by prioritizing essential nutrients, selecting appropriate foods, and maintaining adequate hydration. A personalized approach to diet and hydration, tailored to individual needs and preferences, can help optimize outcomes and improve quality of life for those

CHAPTER 4
DESIGNING A DIET PLAN FOR STIFF PERSON SYNDROME

Designing a Stiff Person Syndrome Diet Plan necessitates a thorough awareness of individual nutritional requirements, balanced meal composition, effective meal planning tactics, and flexibility to accommodate personal preferences and limits.

Assessing Individual Dietary Needs entails a thorough evaluation of the nutritional requirements of individuals diagnosed with Stiff Person Syndrome (SPS), a rare neurological disorder characterized by muscle stiffness and spasms, often accompanied by autoimmune components. Because dietary factors can influence autoimmune conditions and overall health, it's essential to consider a variety of aspects when assessing dietary needs.

Individuals with Stiff Person Syndrome must create balanced meals to optimize their nutritional intake and support overall health and well-being. A balanced meal should provide a variety of nutrients in appropriate proportions, including carbohydrates, proteins, healthy fats, vitamins, and minerals. Carbohydrates are essential for providing energy, and choosing complex carbohydrates such as whole grains, fruits, and vegetables can help stabilize blood sugar.

Setting aside time for meal preparation, creating a weekly menu, compiling a grocery list based on planned recipes, and batch cooking or prepping ingredients are all steps in meal planning, which can help individuals with Stiff Person Syndrome stick to their dietary recommendations consistently.

Adapting the Diet to Personal Preferences and Restrictions acknowledges that dietary recommendations must be tailored to accommodate individual preferences, cultural influences, and dietary restrictions or allergies. While certain guidelines may apply universally for managing Stiff Person Syndrome, such as emphasizing whole, nutrient-dense foods and limiting processed foods high in sugar, salt, and unhealthy fats, there is room for flexibility and customization. For example, individuals with specific food allergies or intolerances may need to avoid certain ingredients or find suitable substitutes. Similarly, cultural preferences and dietary habits should be considered when designing a personalized diet plan to ensure it is culturally relevant and sustainable for the individual. Collaboration between healthcare professionals, such as registered dietitians or nutritionists, and individuals with SPS is essential to develop a diet plan that meets their nutritional needs while accommodating their preferences and restrictions. Regular monitoring and adjustments may be necessary based on changes in health status, symptoms, or lifestyle factors.

CHAPTER 5

EXAMPLE MEAL PLANS FOR STIFF PERSON SYNDROME

For people suffering from Stiff Person Syndrome (SPS), meal planning is crucial for managing symptoms and promoting overall health and well-being. A well-designed meal plan can help alleviate symptoms like muscle stiffness, spasms, and pain while also supporting the body's nutritional needs. A daily meal plan typically includes breakfast, lunch, dinner, and snacks, all carefully curated to provide adequate nutrition and support symptom management.

Breakfast options for SPS patients frequently focus on nutrient-dense foods that provide sustained energy throughout the morning while also being easy to digest. This may include whole grains such as oats or quinoa, which are high in fiber and can help regulate blood sugar levels. Adding protein sources such as eggs, tofu, or Greek yogurt can further enhance satiety and muscle function. Incorporating fruits or vegetables into breakfast can also provide essential vitamins and minerals.

Grilled chicken or fish paired with quinoa or brown rice and a variety of vegetables can provide essential nutrients while also promoting muscle health and function. Lunch meal plans for individuals with SPS frequently revolve around balanced meals that contain a combination of lean proteins, healthy fats, and complex carbohydrates. Adding sources of healthy fats such as avocado, nuts, or olive oil can further enhance the nutritional profile of the meal and support overall

Dinner options for those with SPS may include a similar balance of nutrients as lunch but can vary in composition to provide variety and accommodate individual preferences. Meals centered on lean proteins such as lean beef, turkey, or legumes, paired with whole grains like barley or farro and a variety of colorful vegetables, can provide a satisfying and nourishing dinner. Incorporating herbs, spices, and flavorful sauces can enhance the taste of meals without compromising.

Snacks play an essential role in supporting energy levels and managing hunger throughout the day for individuals with SPS. Optimal snacks are often nutrient-dense and provide a balance of macronutrients to support overall health and well-being. Examples of healthy snacks for SPS patients may include fresh fruit with nut butter, Greek yogurt with granola, or raw vegetables with hummus.

These options provide a combination of carbohydrates, protein, and healthy fats to help stabilize blood sugar levels and promote satiety.

Recipes and meal ideas appropriate for SPS patients:

Incorporating a variety of foods rich in vitamins, minerals, and antioxidants can help alleviate symptoms like muscle stiffness and spasms while also promoting optimal well-being. When developing meal ideas and recipes for people with Stiff Person Syndrome (SPS), it's critical to focus on nutrient-dense ingredients that support symptom management and overall health. Here are some recipes and meal ideas for SPS patients:

1. Quinoa Salad with Grilled Chicken and Vegetables: This nutritious and flavorful salad combines protein-rich grilled chicken breast with fiber-rich quinoa and colorful vegetables like bell peppers, cucumbers, and cherry tomatoes. Tossed with a light vinaigrette dressing of olive oil, lemon juice, and herbs, this meal is both satisfying and nourishing.

2. Baked Salmon with Sweet Potato and Broccoli: This delicious dinner option contains omega-3 fatty acids from baked salmon, which can reduce inflammation and support muscle health. It is also high in vitamins, minerals, and antioxidants, which are important for overall health.

3. Vegetable Stir-Fry with Tofu: This quick and easy stir-fry recipe features a colorful array of vegetables, including bell peppers, snap peas, carrots, and broccoli, sautéed

with tofu for added protein. Seasoned with ginger, garlic, and soy sauce, this flavorful dish is served over brown rice or quinoa for a satisfying and nutritious meal.

4. Turkey and Black Bean Chili: This hearty and comforting chili recipe is packed with lean ground turkey, black beans, tomatoes, and spices such as cumin, chili powder, and paprika. It's loaded with protein, fiber, and essential nutrients, which can help stabilize blood sugar levels and promote muscle health.

5. Greek Yogurt Parfait with Fresh Fruit and Granola: This nutritious and delicious parfait has creamy Greek yogurt, fresh berries, sliced bananas, and crunchy granola.

It's rich in protein, probiotics, and antioxidants, making it a fulfilling and nourishing snack or breakfast option.

Tips For Meal Prep And Cooking Techniques:

Meal preparation and cooking techniques are crucial in creating nutritious and flavorful meals for individuals with Stiff Person Syndrome (SPS).

By incorporating smart strategies and techniques, it is possible to optimize the nutritional value of meals while also enhancing taste and enjoyment. Here are some tips for meal preparation and cooking techniques for SPS patients.

1. Prioritize Whole, Nutrient-Dense Foods: Fruits, vegetables, whole grains, lean proteins, and healthy fats are high in essential nutrients and antioxidants that can alleviate SPS symptoms and promote overall health and well-being.

2. To ensure a varied range of nutrients, include a selection of colored fruits and vegetables in your meals.

Experiment with different textures, such as raw, steaming, roasted, or grilled.

3. Choose lean protein sources like chicken, turkey, fish, tofu, beans, and legumes to support muscle health and function. Trim excess fat and skin from meat to reduce saturated fat intake and promote heart health.

4. Experiment with Herbs and Spices: Use herbs, spices, and aromatics like garlic, ginger, basil, cilantro, cumin, and paprika to add depth and complexity to your meals without adding extra salt or fat.

These ingredients may also provide health benefits.

5. Practice Mindful Eating: Savor and enjoy your meals by paying attention to flavors, textures, and scents.

Techniques include chewing gently, avoiding distractions, and listening to your body's hunger and fullness cues.

6. Streamline meal preparation by planning ahead of time and batch cooking essentials like grains, meats, and veggies.

Pre-cooked ingredients can be stored in the fridge or freezer for simple assembly throughout the week.

7. Use Healthy Cooking Methods: Steaming, sautéing, grilling, roasting, or baking are low-fat cooking methods that retain vitamins, minerals, and antioxidants while increasing flavor.

Individuals with Stiff Person Syndrome (SPS) can create nutritious, flavorful meals that support symptom management and promote overall health and well-being by incorporating these tips and techniques into meal preparation and cooking.

Experiment with different ingredients, flavors, and cooking methods to see what works best for you and your specific dietary needs and preferences.

CHAPTER 6
SPECIAL CONSIDERATIONS AND CHALLENGES

Dealing with Food Intolerances and Allergies: Individuals with Stiff Person Syndrome (SPS) often face the added challenge of managing food intolerances and allergies alongside their primary condition. This necessitates a careful examination of dietary components to identify triggers that may exacerbate symptoms or induce adverse reactions. Food intolerances typically involve difficulty digesting certain substances, such as lactose or gluten, leading to gastrointestinal discomfort, bloating, or other symptoms. Allergies, on the other hand, manifest as immune responses to specific proteins within foods, potentially causing more severe reactions like hives, swelling, or anaphylaxis. Managing these dietary concerns requires meticulous attention to ingredient labels, as well as proactive communication with healthcare providers to develop tailored dietary plans. Elimination diets, where problematic foods are gradually removed and then reintroduced under supervision, can help pinpoint triggers and inform long-term dietary strategies.

Additionally, incorporating alternative ingredients and diversifying food choices can mitigate the risk of nutrient deficiencies while accommodating dietary restrictions. Overall, navigating food intolerances and allergies in the context of SPS demands a comprehensive approach that prioritizes symptom management, nutritional adequacy, and individualized dietary preferences.

Managing Digestive Issues Associated with SPS: Digestive issues often accompany Stiff Person Syndrome (SPS), presenting significant challenges to individuals striving to maintain optimal health and well-being. The neurological abnormalities characteristic of SPS can disrupt the intricate balance of the gastrointestinal system, leading to symptoms such as constipation, diarrhea, abdominal pain, and bloating. These manifestations may stem from the dysregulation of neurotransmitters involved in gut motility and function, highlighting the complex interplay between neurological and digestive processes. Management of digestive issues in SPS necessitates a multifaceted approach encompassing dietary modifications, lifestyle interventions, and pharmacological therapies. Dietary strategies may include incorporating fiber-rich foods to promote regular bowel movements, avoiding trigger foods that exacerbate symptoms, and staying hydrated to support digestive function. Probiotics and prebiotics may also offer benefits by modulating gut microbiota and improving overall gastrointestinal health. Furthermore, stress management techniques and regular physical activity can help alleviate digestive discomfort by reducing tension and promoting relaxation. Collaborative efforts between patients and healthcare providers are essential to tailor interventions according to individual needs and optimize symptom control.

By addressing digestive issues comprehensively, individuals with SPS can enhance their quality of life and mitigate the impact of gastrointestinal symptoms on daily functioning.

Eating Out and Social Situations: Navigating social situations and dining out can pose unique challenges for individuals with Stiff Person Syndrome (SPS), necessitating careful planning and adaptation strategies to ensure enjoyment while managing dietary restrictions and symptom triggers.

Eating out often involves limited control over ingredients and preparation methods, increasing the risk of inadvertently consuming foods that may exacerbate SPS symptoms or trigger adverse reactions.

To mitigate these risks, individuals can employ various strategies, such as researching restaurant menus in advance, communicating dietary needs to restaurant staff, and advocating for modifications to accommodate specific preferences or restrictions.

Choosing restaurants with diverse menu options and flexible customization can offer greater flexibility and ensure a more enjoyable dining experience. Additionally, practicing mindfulness and portion control can help manage symptoms related to SPS while promoting mindful eating habits and satisfaction. Social support networks, including friends, family, and support groups, can provide invaluable encouragement and understanding, fostering a sense of inclusivity and acceptance in social settings. By proactively addressing challenges associated with eating out and social situations, individuals with SPS can enhance their ability to participate in social activities and maintain a balanced approach to nutrition and well-being.

CHAPTER 7

LIFESTYLE STRATEGIES FOR DIETARY MANAGEMENT

Incorporating Physical Activity into the Daily Routine

Physical activity plays a pivotal role in supporting dietary management, particularly for individuals with Stiff Person Syndrome (SPS). Engaging in regular exercise not only aids in weight management but also contributes to overall well-being and functional capacity. For individuals with SPS, tailored exercise routines are imperative to address specific needs and limitations. Low-impact exercises such as walking, swimming, or gentle stretching can help improve flexibility, reduce muscle stiffness, and enhance mobility without exacerbating symptoms. Moreover, incorporating resistance training exercises can strengthen muscles, improve posture, and increase endurance, thereby facilitating better management of SPS symptoms. Individuals with SPS must work closely with healthcare professionals, such as physiotherapists or rehabilitation specialists, to develop personalized exercise regimens that accommodate their unique abilities and limitations. Additionally, integrating physical activity into daily routines, such as taking short walks after meals or incorporating stretching exercises into breaks, can help promote consistency and adherence to an active lifestyle, which is essential for the long-term management of SPS and overall health.

Stress Management Techniques:

The impact of stress on Stiff Person Syndrome (SPS) cannot be overstated, as stress often exacerbates symptoms and negatively affects overall well-being. Therefore, adopting effective stress management techniques is vital for individuals with SPS to enhance their quality of life and support dietary management. Various strategies can be employed to mitigate stress levels, including mindfulness meditation, deep breathing exercises, progressive muscle relaxation, and cognitive-behavioral therapy (CBT). Mindfulness-based practices cultivate present-moment awareness, allowing individuals to observe their thoughts and emotions without judgment, thus reducing stress reactivity and promoting a sense of calmness and inner peace. Similarly, deep breathing exercises, such as diaphragmatic breathing or box breathing, help activate the body's relaxation response, leading to decreased muscle tension and physiological arousal. Additionally, techniques like progressive muscle relaxation involve systematically tensing and releasing muscle groups, promoting physical relaxation and alleviating muscle stiffness associated with SPS. Furthermore, cognitive-behavioral therapy techniques enable individuals to identify and challenge maladaptive thought patterns and behaviors, thereby empowering them to effectively cope with stressors and cultivate resilience.

Integrating these stress management techniques into daily routines can significantly enhance the psychological well-being of individuals with SPS, complementing dietary management efforts and promoting overall health and resilience.

Sleep Hygiene and Its Effect on Nutrition:

Sleep hygiene plays a crucial role in optimizing nutrition and overall health, particularly for individuals with Stiff Person Syndrome (SPS), who may already contend with sleep disturbances due to pain, discomfort, or muscle stiffness. Poor sleep hygiene not only disrupts physiological processes involved in metabolism and appetite regulation but also contributes to mood disturbances, impaired cognitive function, and decreased immune function.

Therefore, prioritizing good sleep hygiene practices is paramount for individuals with SPS to support their dietary management and overall well-being. Establishing a consistent sleep schedule and bedtime routine helps regulate the body's internal clock, promoting better sleep quality and duration. Moreover, creating a sleep-conducive environment by minimizing noise, light, and electronic distractions can enhance sleep onset and maintenance.

Additionally, practicing relaxation techniques before bedtime, such as gentle stretching, progressive muscle relaxation, or meditation, can alleviate muscle tension and promote relaxation, facilitating an easier transition to sleep.

Furthermore, limiting caffeine and alcohol consumption, especially in the evening, and avoiding heavy meals close to bedtime can prevent sleep disturbances and promote better digestion. Adequate hydration is also essential, as dehydration can exacerbate muscle stiffness and discomfort, affecting sleep quality.

By prioritizing good sleep hygiene practices, individuals with SPS can optimize their nutritional status, support dietary management efforts, and promote overall health and well-being.

CHAPTER 8
MONITORING AND ADJUSTING THE DIET PLAN

Monitoring and adjusting the diet plan is an essential aspect of managing Stiff Person Syndrome (SPS), a rare neurological disorder characterized by stiffness, rigidity, and spasms of the muscles. Given the complexity and variability of SPS symptoms among individuals, a personalized approach to diet management is crucial. This section discusses three key concepts: tracking symptoms and dietary intake, working with healthcare professionals, and making necessary adjustments to optimize results.

Tracking Symptoms and Dietary Intake: Because individuals with SPS frequently experience fluctuating symptoms that may be influenced by various factors, including diet, keeping a detailed record of symptoms and dietary intake is paramount in understanding potential triggers and patterns.

Working with Healthcare Professionals: Collaborating with healthcare professionals, including registered dietitians, neurologists, and other specialists familiar with SPS, is vital for developing and implementing an effective dietary management plan. These professionals can offer valuable expertise in understanding the interplay between nutrition and SPS symptoms, interpreting dietary records, and recommending evidence-based dietary interventions tailored to individual needs. Moreover, they can conduct comprehensive assessments to identify potential nutrient deficiencies or metabolic abnormalities associated with SPS and guide appropriate dietary modifications or supplementation strategies to address these issues.

Furthermore, healthcare professionals play a crucial role in coordinating interdisciplinary care and facilitating communication between the individual, caregivers, and other members of the healthcare team to ensure holistic management of SPS.

Making Necessary Adjustments to Optimize Results: As the effectiveness of dietary interventions may vary among individuals with SPS, ongoing monitoring and adjustment of the diet plan are essential to optimize outcomes. This entails a systematic approach to evaluating the impact of dietary changes on symptom management and overall well-being and making necessary adjustments based on observed outcomes and feedback from healthcare professionals. For instance, if certain foods consistently exacerbate symptoms or if nutrient deficiencies are identified, modifications to the diet plan may be warranted, such as eliminating trigger foods, adjusting macronutrient ratios, or incorporating specific nutrient-rich foods or supplements. Additionally, factors such as changes in medication regimens, comorbidities, and lifestyle factors should be considered when refining the diet plan to ensure comprehensive management of SPS. By continually assessing and adapting the diet plan in response to individual needs and evolving circumstances, individuals with SPS can optimize symptom control, improve nutritional status, and enhance overall quality of life.

In summary, monitoring and adjusting the diet plan are integral components of managing Stiff Person Syndrome.

By tracking symptoms and dietary intake, collaborating with healthcare professionals, and making necessary adjustments to optimize results, individuals with SPS can effectively manage symptoms, address nutritional needs, and improve overall well-being. Individuals with SPS can empower themselves through a personalized and proactive approach to dietary management.

CHAPTER 9

RESOURCES AND ADDITIONAL SUPPORT

Online Community and Support Groups:

Individuals with Stiff Person Syndrome (SPS) and seeking dietary guidance can benefit greatly from online communities and support groups. These virtual spaces provide a platform for individuals to share their experiences, exchange information, and offer emotional support. Participating in such communities can foster a sense of belonging and reduce feelings of isolation that are often experienced by those with chronic conditions like SPS.

Recommended Books And Websites:

Accessing reliable information is essential for individuals managing SPS, and there are numerous recommended books and websites that offer valuable insights into personalized dietary approaches for optimal health and well-being. Books authored by healthcare professionals specializing in nutrition and autoimmune disorders can provide in-depth knowledge about dietary interventions, meal planning, and lifestyle strategies tailored to managing SPS symptoms. These resources often include evidence-based information, practical tips, and recipe suggestions to help individuals make informed decisions about their dietary choices. Additionally, reputable websites curated by healthcare organizations, patient advocacy groups, and nutrition experts offer a wealth of information on SPS, including dietary guidelines, research updates, and links to relevant studies. These platforms serve as reliable sources of information and empower individuals to take an active role in managing their condition through dietary interventions.

Accessing Professional Nutritional Counseling:

Seeking professional nutritional counseling is paramount for individuals with SPS to develop personalized dietary plans that address their specific needs and goals. Registered dietitians (RDs) specializing in autoimmune disorders can provide tailored nutritional guidance based on individual health profiles, medical history, and dietary preferences. These professionals possess expertise in assessing nutrient requirements, identifying potential dietary triggers, and recommending appropriate dietary modifications to alleviate symptoms and promote overall well-being. Through comprehensive nutritional assessments, RDs can help individuals with SPS optimize their nutrient intake, manage weight, and address any nutrient deficiencies or imbalances that may exacerbate symptoms. Moreover, nutritional counseling sessions may include education on label reading, meal planning strategies, and practical tips for navigating social situations and dining out while adhering to dietary restrictions. By collaborating with a qualified RD, individuals with SPS can gain valuable insights and support to implement sustainable dietary changes that support their health and quality of life.

CONCLUSION

adopting a personalized dietary approach is crucial for individuals living with Stiff Person Syndrome (SPS) to manage symptoms, optimize health, and enhance overall well-being. By understanding the underlying mechanisms of SPS and its potential impact on nutritional status, individuals can make informed dietary choices that alleviate symptoms, support immune function, and promote neuroprotection. A holistic approach to dietary management may involve identifying and eliminating potential trigger foods, optimizing nutrient intake, and implementing lifestyle strategies to reduce inflammation and oxidative stress.

Through collaboration with healthcare professionals, including registered dietitians specializing in autoimmune disorders, individuals with SPS can develop personalized dietary plans tailored to their unique needs and preferences.

Moreover, accessing online communities, recommended books, and professional nutritional counseling can provide additional support and resources to empower individuals in their journey toward optimal health and well-being.

By integrating dietary interventions into comprehensive management strategies, individuals with SPS can enhance their quality of life and cultivate resilience in the face of this chronic neurological condition.

Made in the USA
Las Vegas, NV
27 May 2024

90449492R00035